The ADHD Guide for Parents

Tips on How to Help Your Child Improve Attention, Manage Emotions and Achieve Goals

By: Rose McCloud

9781681275116

PUBLISHERS NOTES

Disclaimer – Speedy Publishing LLC

This publication is intended to provide helpful and informative material. It is not intended to diagnose, treat, cure, or prevent any health problem or condition, nor is intended to replace the advice of a physician. No action should be taken solely on the contents of this book. Always consult your physician or qualified health-care professional on any matters regarding your health and before adopting any suggestions in this book or drawing inferences from it.

The author and publisher specifically disclaim all responsibility for any liability, loss or risk, personal or otherwise, which is incurred as a consequence, directly or indirectly, from the use or application of any contents of this book.

Any and all product names referenced within this book are the trademarks of their respective owners. None of these owners have sponsored, authorized, endorsed, or approved this book.

Always read all information provided by the manufacturers' product labels before using their products. The author and publisher are not responsible for claims made by manufacturers.

This book was originally printed before 2014. This is an adapted reprint by Speedy Publishing LLC with newly updated content designed to help readers with much more accurate and timely information and data.

Speedy Publishing LLC

40 E Main Street, Newark, Delaware, 19711

Contact Us: 1-888-248-4521

Website: http://www.speedypublishing.co

REPRINTED Paperback Edition: 9781681275116:

Manufactured in the United States of America

Dedication

This book is dedicated to Theodore. You are my heaven on earth. Regardless of how big you get and how old you will be, you will always be in my heart.

TABLE OF CONTENTS

Chapter 1- ADHD and Its Effects on Your Child 5

Chapter 2- Diagnosing ADD under ADHD 10

Chapter 3- What's the Best Treatment for Your Child? 18

Chapter 4- Can Hypnosis Help? 22

Chapter 5- Hypnosis as a Physical Treatment 30

Chapter 6- Training Children with ADHD/ADD for Success 36

Chapter 7- What's It Like Living with ADHD/ADD? 43

About The Author 47

CHAPTER 1- ADHD AND ITS EFFECTS ON YOUR CHILD

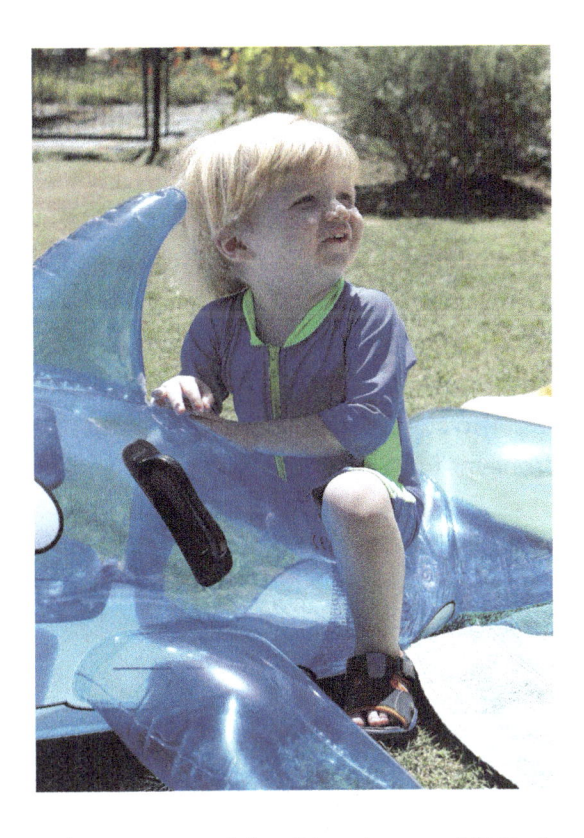

Attention Deficit Hyperactivity Disorder or ADHD is a mental disorder, which approximately three to seven percent children are having. Due to this disorder children manifest the characteristic of constant behavior, loads of activity as well as often being considered disobedient. That does not mean that the individual is being bad but the thing is they don't have control over their mental range. They go through lack of concentration because at a time they are likely to be thinking about many elements instead of one particular element.

This disorder is also found in many adults besides children. In adults, it is called Adult Attention Deficit Disorder or AADD. Among all children diagnosed with ADHD about 30 to 70 percent will carry

The ADHD and ADD Guide for Parents

on with their disorder through adulthood. Adults learn to live with it and work around it and need less help. They can handle the disorder of their own and so it's harder to detect also. Yet, in many cases both children and adult may need medications for better results.

In children this disorder shows signs like inattentiveness, impulsive behavior and a constant restlessness. In adults, it is harder to diagnose but children with this disorder cannot sit still for long. They cannot concentrate on one particular thing for a long period of time. In adults, it becomes difficult sometimes to structure their lives and to plan daily activities. They don't feel the importance to stay attentive or to stop being restless because these are not at all important problems for them.

ADHD is a disorder for which assistance of medical personnel is necessary. It can be treated but cannot be cured fully. For this disorder medication is also necessary.

The 5 Types of ADHD

Attention Deficit Hyperactivity Disorder has many manifestations and there are more than five kinds of ADHD. It is a medical condition that is carried in the genes, resulting in certain disorders in the nervous system.

The DSM-IV Diagnostic Manual reports that any single form or "type" of Attention Deficit Hyperactivity Disorder could be categorized under the diagnostic chapter of ADHD. This central list is then broken into ADHD Impulsive-Hyperactive Type, ADHD Inattentive Type, or ADHD Combined Type. Sometime ago, the words attention deficit disorder "without" or "with" hyperactivity were also generally used. Not only does the Attention Deficit Hyperactivity can take various forms, but also there could be so suggest that approximately 4.4% of all adults possess some degree of ADD.

ADD is understood as a disorder of the neurobiological type caused in brain by a glitch in the dopamine neurotransmitter systems. Genes play a huge part in maximum cases. There is 30% chance for a child to have ADD if a parent or near kith and kin has the disorder. In twins; if one has ADD then the other's chances of being struck by the disease increases by 50%. At one time the belief was held that ADD could be caused by poor nutrition, but it has been dismissed now as a myth. Similarly, allergies, drugs or bad parenting could be cut off from the list. Deep head trauma, fetal alcohol syndrome, intoxication through lead, and thyroid irregularities, are some of the other medical conditions showing symptoms like ADD. Hence it is advised that the other possibilities are rules out completely before the person could be said to have ADD for sure.

Having ADD means that an individual having it is not getting sufficient neuro-chemicals. Said in simpler terms it signifies that proper stimulation of the brain is missing, as a result of which the brain attempts to find methods by which the release of the chemicals can be increased. People with ADD try to stimulate their brains with things like physical activities, movements, and always doing things that stimulate or are stimulating. This is not a conscious decision on the parts of the people with ADD. They really cannot help themselves and it becomes a reflex action and they act in a hyperactive manner.

The difficulty caused by this is that individuals who suffer from ADD, when face a circumstance that do not stimulate them, like school work, try to put their attention on something that is stimulating to them. Of course the school work is completely hampered by this, and the child cannot perform well in his or her studies. I can narrate a story here told to me by a friend. This incident happened when knowledge about the disease was poor. There was a child who would suddenly get up on his desk when the class is still commencing, and would begin to tell jokes. In the beginning people thought that he was trying to be funny and consciously disturb the others. But over time it came to be known that the child had ADD, and his actions were beyond his control.

Personal relationships and the ability to be permanently employed also become cause of concern for people with ADD. Then legal issue also crop up when ADD causes people to take dangerous chances with themselves and end up doing careless things to stimulate themselves.

ADHD vs. ADD

Attention Deficit Disorder or ADD is a very complicated, and time and again misinterpreted, disorder. Its beginning is physiological, but it can have a multitude of consequences that come alongside with it. That apart, what is the differentiation between ADHD and ADD? ADHD is the abbreviated form of Attention Deficit Hyperactive Disorder, its major indications being noticeable hyperactivity and impulsivity. These are the indications that are noticeable to the purposeful onlooker. ADD stands for Attention Deficit Disorder with the major indications being lack of concentration. Now a lot of other things can come alongside with both of these subtypes of ADHD, but those are the distinctive characteristics of both.

For several years, the usual picture of Attention Deficit Disorder has been the little boy that is bouncing off the walls and making his teachers and parents go mad. ADHD is beyond a doubt the more identifiable of the two subtypes since it is so much more noticeable than ADD. Since hyperactivity causes a lot more disruption and problems for classrooms, it gets the most notice and will be picked up on a lot quicker. Unluckily, even if ADD is less visible, the consequences of the disorder can just as negative.

With negligent attention deficit disorder, or ADD, the person enduring it will give the impression of being spacey and disordered. More often, victims with this type will be gazing out of the window during classes and will seem as if they are never somewhat there. It is much trickier to make a diagnosis and a lot of people with this form of ADD go years without even knowing they have it. But the consequences of the drifting mind can be just as disparaging.

For a long time, it was considered that only boys suffered from ADHD. However, this figment has been busted of late. It is now acknowledged that both girls and boys can suffer from attention deficit disorder, and many do not get out of it in middle age. One disparity that has been noticed is that girls are inclined to have the inattentive version of ADD, and many times it is wrongly diagnosed as depression. Since inattentive ADD does not create noticeable troubles and disruptions to the nearby surroundings, a lot of them endure in silence for years before they discover the real reason of their plight.

With both ADHD and ADD, making a diagnosis early on is very essential. Even though troubles with schools are the most apparent indications, some victims do not have major problems with getting school work completed. Keep track of your children, not just academically, but generally and psychologically as well. Do they have problem with other children? Does it appear as if they have difficulty putting in order or are extremely disordered? Do they have difficulty sitting motionless for a period of time? Are they extremely silent or extremely chatty? Now any of these indications do not in particular denote ADD or ADHD, but they do point to asking for outside help from a therapist or a counselor.

The ADHD and ADD Guide for Parents

Your child's psychological wellbeing is just as vital as their physical wellbeing and how they do in school. Confirm it out if you sense like something is off. If left for years not diagnosed, ADD can create a lot of other resulting troubles that can take a long time to get rid of and can be arrested.

Reading Symptoms in Children

Attention Deficit Disorder can take several forms in children. It is not difficult to track the child with ADD who is very chaotic. Boys generally come into this category. But then there are some types of ADD which go undiagnosed because their effects in children are less outwardly evident. This happens mainly in case of girls.

There are many girls who are called "tomboys". They frequently exhibit some of the important features off ADD, like being more involved in physical activities, but not as reckless as the boys themselves. As a result teachers and parents jump to the conclusion that the child has no interest in academics and is basically not organized, but the possibility of ADD is seldom considered.

Besides the "tomboy" types, the "chatty" girls could also be suffering from ADD, but remaining undiagnosed. This is a fusion of over-activity and inattentiveness, and is usually touted as socially extrovert. These girls are extremely talkative than being physically active and cannot stop talking even if they are strictly warned. They also cannot tell stories comprehensively and will stray from their thoughts because of ADD.

Those whom we call as "daydreamers" could also be suffering from ADD. They do not draw any attention to themselves and are very quiet in nature. However, their too much being into themselves and not giving any attention to the class is another form of ADD, contrary to the "chatty" girls. They may show anxiety and depression when given school projects, but cannot finish the projects because of their lack of staying power. This generally goes undiagnosed because the child is thought to be lazy and, parents and teachers fail to identify the disorder in time.

What is fascinating is that many girls with ADD have quite a high rate of IQ and could be called "gifted". When a child has a high IQ there are no problems in school work, but their lack loopholes get reflected as they mature into adults. Keep in mind that ADD is not a learning disorder, and patients do not inevitably are poor performers in school. Till high school they can be quite well off, but with mounting pressure and assignments symptoms may become more and more evident.

When undiagnosed, Attention Deficit Disorder may cause a lot of harm to an individual. Children will be called unorganized, lacking intelligence and lazy, when in truth, they might be silent sufferers of ADD. They will have very low esteem of themselves, and believe themselves to be quitters or stupid because of their problems. It is crucial that the problem is identifies and treated before it becomes too late and any long-term damage is done.

Coming Up with a Diagnosis

Assessing whether a certain individual is suffering from Attention Deficit Disorder or not is far harder than it appears to laymen like us. This is because, not only does it's symptoms largely overlap those of hyperthyroidism etc. they are also largely exhibited by 'normal' human beings some time or the other every single day. Therefore the first important step towards diagnosing the disease is to consult a trained health care provider regarding it.

Given that the defining factors of Attention Deficit Disorder is still quite musty and vague diagnosing the problem is difficult since nothing is strictly within or outside the peripheries of the disease. And although various organizations like The American Pediatrics Clinical Practice for instance, have tried to provide certain guidelines in order to recognize the disease most are still quite unsure regarding the reliability of such methods. Of course doctors have in the past tried MRI (or magnetic resonance imagery) to analyze their patient's brains in order to detect any possible signs of ADD, but most medical practitioners do not recommend this anymore. Thus diagnosis is now primarily based on the reports of those close to the patient, who see, talk, work or live with him/her every day and have thereby come to know the patients habits closely. A number of people suffering from ADD also realize their problem with time, especially as they grow older and consult doctors regarding it.

The guideline provided by the American Academy of pediatrics requires medical personnel to look into the child's behavior in more than one place before reaching a conclusion regarding whether or not the child is suffering from ADD. Thus the doctor is expected to consult various 'witnesses' regarding the behavior of his patient in say his school, his home, at the playground, at his Grandma's place etc. and thereby ensure that his diagnosis is not based on the child's behavior at a certain specific place. This is to know for sure that the problem in hand is intrinsic and is consistent everywhere and not specifically due to some factors at a particular place. The guideline also requires the physician to use an "explicit criteria for the diagnosis using the DS-IV-TR".

When approaching a doctor for cure therefore make sure that he/she follows these directions set by the Academy closely before diagnosing the problem. Remember a problem such as ADD might

Rose McCloud

not be as difficult to cure as to diagnose, in fact proper diagnosis might be the first step towards a satisfactory cure.

ADD is an underestimated disease which is seen in varying degrees amongst many youngsters around us and while we may choose to ignore it and deny it's presence it's a plague which will follow your little one right till he shuts his eyes for good. Therefore recognize your child's disease today and take him to a doctor for the right diagnosis and a proper cure.

Chapter 3 - What's the Best Treatment for Your Child?

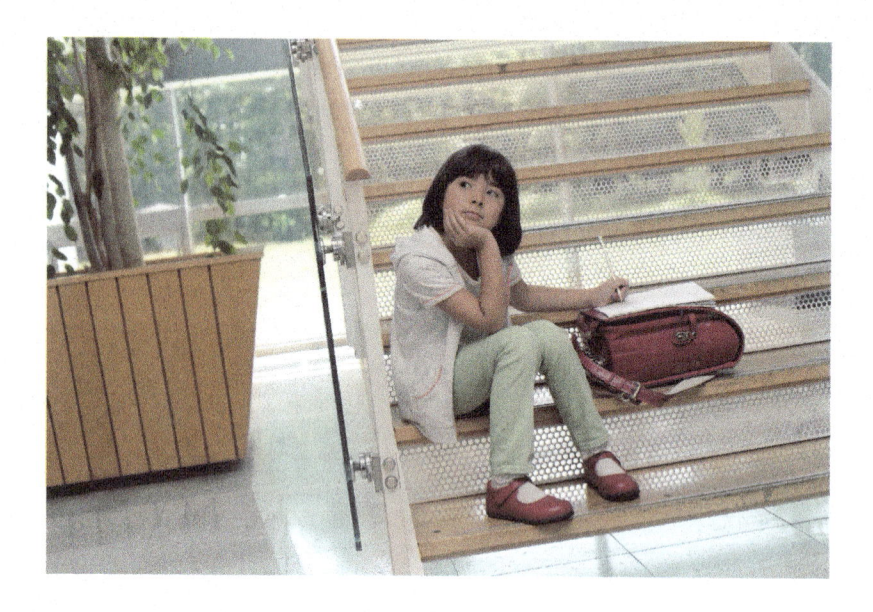

Okay. So at the moment you have taken the action of getting your stressed-out child or teenager evaluated by an expert, and he has been identified with Attention Deficit Hyperactivity Disorder. The psychologist, or therapist, or physician now desires to start a healing course. But what are you supposed to know before you "sign off" on any specific healing plan?

Here are some propositions for you to think about. Given below are purely our propositions, but are founded on having worked with more than 1,000 children and teenagers with attention deficit hyperactivity disorder. Make use of your best opinion. Have a discussion with your doctor. We do not want to be blamed of practicing medicine over the Internet. The diagnoses that come along will differ based on your child or teen's analysis.

All through the summer holiday and near the beginning of the school year we like to attempt the "alternative" involvements, such as homeopathy, our suggested eating plan, and necessary fatty acid supplements. EEG Biofeedback training is also a fine "alternative" healing for ADD. If these approaches are effective, and they will around 70% of the time, then we can keep the patient away from medicines and observe them do well.

If the analysis is made later on in the school year we have a tendency to propose tryouts of medicine right away for just about each one with Attention Deficit Disorder, aware that we have the summer coming up to attempt options that may be able to reduce the dosage of medicine in half, or do away with the requirement for medicine all in all. But later on in the school year time turn out to be a larger issue. We do not wish for the school year to be used up or lost, so we have to try the most forceful involvements at that time.

But here are our thoughts. Initially we would like to do what we are capable of to "salvage" the school year if we just have a few weeks left. Since medicines can start on to give improvements very swiftly, frequently the child will get through classes that he or she might have failed in another case. In addition, by having a "real world" tryout of medicine ahead of the summer holiday, we can use the advantages got from the medicine as a "bench mark" with which to determine the efficiency of the "alternative" healing that may be tried during the summer months.

Also, please keep in mind when talking about these propositions with your psychologist or your medical doctor, that ancient saying, "If the one tool that you have is a hammer, then all the world looks like a nail." Specialists, who are not familiar with healing alternatives like the EEG Biofeedback training or the "Attend" amino acids, will have a tendency to mark them down straight away out of their lack of knowledge. I did this myself for years, and this is where you have got to come to a decision on yourself how best to lend a hand to your child or teenager with Attention Deficit Disorder.

Available Alternative Treatments for ADD

Given that so many would to a certain extent keep away from the use of stimulant medications for the healing of attention deficit hyperactivity disorder if probable, an increasing want for the growth of alternative treatments for ADD, ADHD has risen since the past twenty years. Even though there are many products that state to help out any child with ADD or ADHD, the fact is that there are only a small amount of non-medicine healing for attention deficit disorder that have in reality gone through even the easiest of medical tests. The majority of alternative healings have never been cautiously studied to find out their efficiency in the real world.

Our four preferred non medicinal healings for attention deficit disorder have been studied in the real world. They are Brainwave Biofeedback training, Behavior Modification therapy, Eating or Diet Interventions, and the Nutraceutical medicines called "Extress" and "Attend".

Therapy can have helpful advantages under some situations, such as the expertise of the counselor in working with ADD or ADHD persons. A lot of counselors have little knowledge in working with these people.

"Attend" and "Extress" are superb substitutes to treatment stimulant medicines. They are very complicated procedures, engineered to achieve maximum efficiency in brain functioning in individuals going through problems with concentration, impulse control, rage, listening attentively, or hyper activity.

Rose McCloud

EEG Biofeedback training, also known as Neurofeedback is around a twenty year old technology. With the ongoing progress of faster and faster computers it has developed into a feasible alternative healing for ADD. There is a vast amount of study on EEG Biofeedback, which you ought to go through if you are at all concerned. The EEG Spectrum is a great web site for a lot of information on this treatment alternative.

Eating plans, or diet involvements, might also have some constructive effect on persons with attention deficit hyperactivity disorder. Even though we do not feel that this involvement is as effectual as either the Attend and Extress, or EEG Biofeedback training, we do consider that every person with ADHD ought to try a diet involvement.

A lot of persons with ADD or ADHD will also be helped from nutritional supplements. The most effectual are most likely Essential Fatty Acids which are also known as Omega Oils and particular minerals like Zinc. The necessary fatty acids you will find present in the "Attend" nutraceutical. You also get them in Borage Oil or Flax Seed Oil. They can in addition be found in fish, and you can just give your child more of tuna fish to eat.

Chapter 4- Can Hypnosis Help?

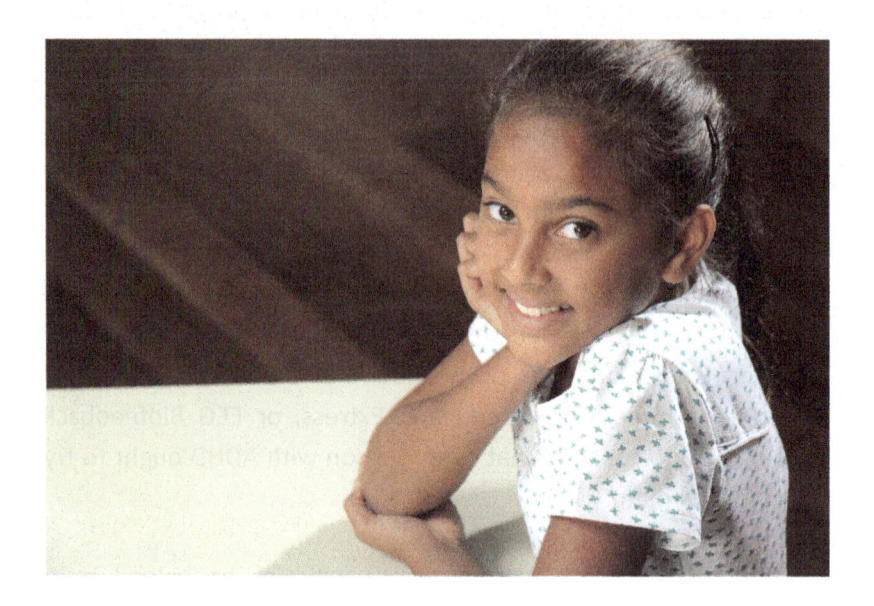

In the most simplistic terms hypnosis can be described as an altered state of consciousness. Most people think of hypnosis as being in a trance like state, but that's not really an accurate description. When you're in a hypnotic state you are really in a super-relaxed state of mind where your conscious mind is so relaxed that you're not thinking at all about normal everyday things. Being hypnotized allows you to connect with your subconscious mind and pull up memories, experiences, and other events that played a significant role in your life or in your development.

Usually a hypnotic state is induced by a trained therapist or medical professional but there are courses that you can take that will teach you how to hypnotize yourself. If you are going to try hypnosis for medical treatment you might want to get a professional to start the treatment and then if they work for you learn how to hypnotize yourself so that you can continue the treatment on your own whenever your condition flares up. While you are in a hypnotic state the therapist or medical professional will create what is called a hypnotic suggestion. The hypnotic suggestion is what tells your subconscious what to change.

So for example if you are being hypnotized to help you deal with your alcohol addiction a hypnotic suggestion telling your brain that you no longer need alcohol to function combined with physical treatment for the withdrawal symptoms that you'll experience when you stop drinking should make you entirely free of alcohol dependency. Your body will no longer crave it once you have detoxed and after a hypnotic suggestion telling you that you don't need the alcohol your mind won't be convinced that you can't function with it.

Doctors aren't entirely sure how the brain creates a hypnotic state only that a hypnotic state exists and can be induced in most people. Hypnotic suggestions aren't an easy fix to medical problems, and many times using hypnosis for medical treatments requires several sessions in order to be fully effective. But there is a growing amount of evidence that using hypnosis to treat hard to treat conditions, especially the kind of medical conditions that have psychological components, can be a very effective way to help an individual create lasting changes in his or her life that will improve health and wellness.

Conditions that don't seem to respond to other treatments usually respond well to hypnotic treatment. If you don't really approve of Western medicine or if you just prefer a more holistic approach to your health care you can try using hypnosis to treat everything from Asthma to pain caused by medical procedures like bone marrow biopsies, Breast Cancer treatment and wound cleaning and stitching. For people that are highly susceptible to hypnosis sometimes hypnosis can even replace anesthesia that would typically knock a patient out during surgery. It's not common practice to hypnotize someone before surgery but for people that

The ADHD and ADD Guide for Parents

have had bad reactions to anesthesia medications hypnosis is one option.

Is Hypnosis for Everyone?

One of the most frequently asked questions when it comes to Hypnosis is whether or not everyone can be hypnotized. Some people are adamant that they can't be hypnotized and are convinced that hypnosis will never work for them. So what's the real answer? Is it impossible for some people to be hypnotized the way that they claim? The answer is yes, and no. Everyone can be hypnotized, theoretically, so there's no physical reason why everyone can't be put into a hypnotic state. But there may be psychological reasons that someone is resistant to being hypnotized which might make it very difficult for that person to relax enough to enter a true hypnotic state.

Usually people who are certain that they can't be hypnotized have a deep seated need for control and think that if they allow themselves to be hypnotized they will be giving up control so they will never allow themselves to relax enough to get to the hypnotic state. But you never give up control of your mind or body during hypnosis and you're never unconscious. Your conscious mind is just very deeply relaxed and letting the subconscious mind come to the forefront. So people that are very sure that can't be hypnotized really can be hypnotized but not until they let go of their belief that being hypnotized means giving up control of themselves to someone else.

Another reason that people have trouble entering a hypnotic state is the particular therapist that they are working with. In order to be able to relax in the very deep way that is necessary in order to become hypnotized it's critical that the person being hypnotized trust the therapist implicitly. If there is any discomfort or mistrust on the part of the person that is being hypnotized he or she will not be able to relax enough to get into the hypnotic state and the treatment won't work.

So when it comes to hypnosis medical experts and psychotherapists along with alternative health practitioners agree that everyone can be hypnotized, but not everyone wants to be. Wanting to be hypnotized and being open to the hypnotic process is very important. It's also important that the person who is going to be hypnotizes feels comfortable with the person doing the hypnotizing. So if you go to a psychologist or an alternative health practitioner to get help to stop smoking but you are uncomfortable with that therapist in any way then it won't work. That therapist won't be able to hypnotize you.

Because of that finding the right hypnotherapist for you, someone that you feel totally comfortable with, is extremely important. Later on we'll look at how you will know which hypnotherapist is right for you and what you should ask a hypnotherapist before you start treatment with that person to make sure that the therapist is well trained, experienced, legitimate, and right for you.

Will It Work on Children?

Hypnotherapy is often used to treat children that have behavioral disorders and children that have had traumatic events happen to them. Children have also been put into a hypnotic state in order to help police solve crimes in crimes where children have been attacked. Some Hypnotherapists have found that using hypnosis as a method of treating night terrors for children under 10 years old can be more effective than other treatments because putting the children in a deep hypnotic state before bed relaxes their brain enough that they don't have night terrors. If your child is having

The ADHD and ADD Guide for Parents

night terrors and has not responded well to other treatments using hypnosis is an option you should discuss with your doctor.

Top Benefits of Health Hypnosis

So how can hypnosis really help you? What are the benefits of going through hypnosis? Those are the questions that most people ask when they first consider going to see a hypnotherapist. Because Hypnosis is considered an unconventional treatment in the West some people are a little apprehensive about considering it as a treatment. But when you think about these benefits that can come from Hypnosis you'll see it's really worth it:

1. Hypnosis can treat addictions – Food, alcohol, drugs, smoking, it doesn't matter what you're addicted to Hypnosis can help you kick the addiction. Hypnosis combined with physical treatment to get rid of your body's physical addition to whatever you are addicted to is proven to help break addictions for good so that you don't relapse and become addicted again within a short time.

2. Hypnosis can help you lose weight and keep it off – Sounds too good to be true right? But it's not. Hypnosis has been proven to be 30% more effective than just dieting when it comes to weight loss. Medical professionals speculate that Hypnosis helps people who are hanging onto the extra weight for psychological reasons or people that overeat for psychological reasons eliminate their psychological need for extra fat or extra food which makes it easier for them to lose weight.

3. Hypnosis can help manage chronic pain – If you have a disease that leaves you in frequent pain like Fibromyalgia or Arthritis then you already knows that sometimes it feels like nothing will stop the pain. When drugs and diet don't help you manage your

pain Hypnosis can. In many different scientific studies Hypnosis has been proven as an effective pain management technique. So if nothing else is working for you when it comes to controlling your pain, or if you don't want to take prescription painkillers, you should try Hypnosis.

4. Hypnosis can help reduce stress – Stress is more than just annoyance. Stress can cause serious illness in people like heart disease, high blood pressure, obesity, diabetes, and sleep disorders. If you have a lot of stress in your life and you feel like you can't get it under control by using diet and exercise then it's time to think about Hypnosis. Because Hypnosis involves putting you in a deep state of relaxation it gives your mind and body a chance to experience the relaxation that they desperately need.

5. Hypnosis can help deal with childhood issues – Childhood issues. Everyone has them. From serious abuse or other problems in the home to lack of self-esteem or a need to be successful at all costs the issues and problems that you experienced as a child might still be impacting you today and causing you to make bad decisions or to not take very good care of yourself. Hypnosis is a great way to work through childhood issues and replace those negative messages about you with positive ones.

6. Hypnosis can cure sleep disorders – Millions of people suffer from sleep disorders that range from full insomnia to night terrors, wakeful sleep, sleepwalking, and the inability to fall into REM sleep which your body needs. Sleep disorders can cause a wide range of other problems like obesity and addiction to either sleeping medications or to caffeine or other stimulants in an effort to keep the body going even though it's exhausted.

Sleep disorders are notoriously hard to treat. Many sleep disorders have an associated psychological condition that makes it necessary for people to get both psychological and physical treatment in order to be able to get some sleep. Hypnosis can help treat the psychological problem that is causing the sleep disturbance while at the same time it puts the body in a deeply relaxed state that helps the body and mind become rejuvenated.

7. Hypnosis can promote deep relaxation – If you have ever tried meditation you know already the great things that relaxation does for the mind and body. You can become more creative, better at problem solving, less irritable, and you can reduce your risk of health problems like heart disease or high blood pressure significantly if you meditate or relax regularly.

But if you have trouble relaxing, or if you never seem to be able to relax deeply enough to really feel refreshed, then you should try Hypnosis. Hypnosis is a wonderful way to experience truly deep relaxation that will make you feel much healthier.

8. Hypnosis can help you change your behavior – Are you the kind of person that is always snapping at others? Do you get irritated and angry often? Do you have trouble managing your anger? Hypnosis can help you change your behavior patterns so that you can be healthier and happier.

Often behavioral patterns are learned in childhood, but a hypnotic suggestion given while you're in a deep hypnotic state can help you get rid of those old messages telling you to behave in certain ways and replace them with messages to act in new, more appropriate ways. If you are trying to recover from the effects of a dysfunctional family or an abusive childhood using Hypnosis to help eliminate the unhealthy patterns that you learned to survive can be very therapeutic.

9. Hypnosis can help recover buried memories – All of the experiences that you've had throughout your life are buried in your brain somewhere. If you have lost touch with the parts of your brain that hold memories of your childhood Hypnosis can help you go back and remember the things that you need to remember in order to know why you act the way you act now. Typically this is used to help people that were abused as children understand their behavioral patterns but there can also be happy memories that you have forgotten as a result of an injury or accident that can be recovered with Hypnosis.

10. Hypnosis can help treat Anxiety and Depression – Many people are reluctant to take medication to treat Anxiety and Depression because they don't want to become dependent on medication. Other people just can't seem to find a medication that works for them. Hypnosis is a drug free and very effective way to calm Anxiety and to treat the symptoms of depression. By using hypnotic suggestions to eliminate the triggers of Anxiety and Depression people that suffer from Depression and Anxiety can sometimes find 100% relief from those conditions by using Hypnosis.

Chapter 5 - Hypnosis as a Physical Treatment

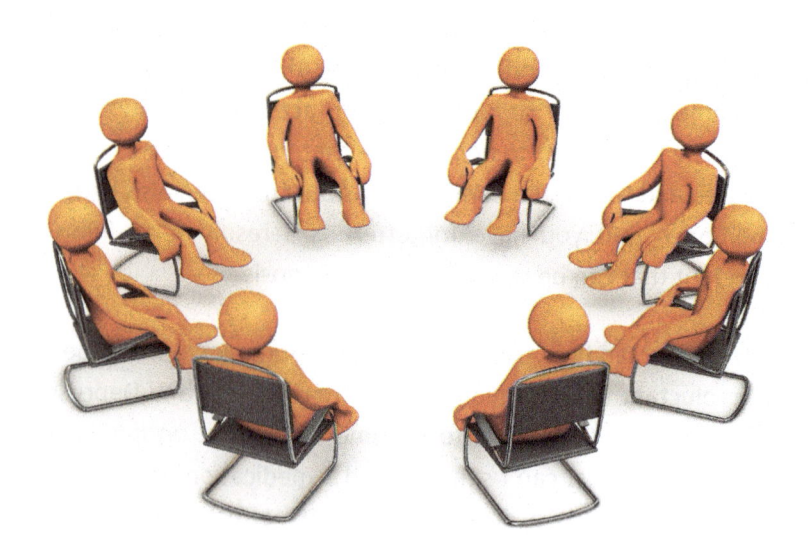

Eastern medicine has recognized the connection between body and mind for a long time. The centuries old Ayurvedic health system in India was built on the principle that anything that is physically wrong with the body has a mental or emotional cause and that in order to treat the physical symptom the emotional or psychological cause had to be cured first.

You might be surprised by how many disorders that are usually treated with drug therapy can also be treated, successfully, with hypnosis. If you or someone that you know suffers from any of these conditions but has not responded well to drug therapy, or is reluctant to try drug therapy because of the fear of side effects or the fear of getting addicted hypnosis is a good option when it comes to treating these disorders:

- Addictions

- Obesity

- Phobias

- Anxiety

- Depression

- OCD

- ADD/ADHD

- Insomnia

- Stress

- Anger Issues

- Childhood Issues

- Sexual Dysfunctions

- Eating Disorders

- Compulsions

Even though medical professionals have never denied the existence of hypnosis they have only begun to embrace hypnosis as a treatment for medical conditions in the past few decades. Hypnosis has been used primarily to treat psychological conditions until the recent past when the medical community began to realize that using hypnosis to treat physical conditions under certain conditions was very effective. In clinical studies, hypnosis was found to be a powerful treatment for some conditions that are very difficult or dangerous to treat with drugs like chronic pain, chronic

The ADHD and ADD Guide for Parents

fatigue, addictions, and even the pain and anxiety associated with childbirth.

Unlike more traditional types of treatment hypnosis is not usually used as a standalone treatment for medical conditions. Instead it's used in conjunction with other therapies to boost the effectiveness of the other therapies and to treat any psychological disorder that might be an underlying cause of the physical problem. The more that Western doctors begin to accept a more holistic idea of medicine and realize that the body and mind are connected so that what affects the body also affects the mind and vice versa the more hypnosis is valued as a treatment for common medical conditions.

Because there are no side effects associated with hypnosis as a medical treatment most doctors, even the ones that don't believe in the power of hypnosis to heal, would not discourage their patients from using it because there's no risk to them to try it.

But more and more clinical studies are being done that prove that hypnosis does work in almost all cases, on all different kinds of people. Western patients are turning more and more to alternative therapies for health care because they don't trust Western doctors, and they don't trust big drug companies and they want treatments that they feel are safe and effective. Hypnosis is the safest type of treatment for many conditions because it has no side effects.

Hypnosis is also a safer treatment than many drug therapies because there is no risk of a bad drug interaction or an allergic reaction to hypnosis. Anyone can be hypnotized regardless of their current health status, allergies, or what medications they are on. If you look at just some of the ways that hypnosis has been used to treat physical conditions you might be surprised at how many different conditions can be treated with hypnosis. Hypnosis can:

- Get rid of the psychological causes of addiction and lessen physical cravings

- Ease withdrawal symptoms

- Eliminate the pain of childbirth

- Manage or eliminate the symptoms of Depression and Anxiety

- Manage pain without drugs in medical surgeries or during dental treatments. This is highly effective for people that have a dental phobia that prevents them from getting routine dental care.

- Treat and eliminate the symptoms of irritable bowel syndrome (IBS)

- Lower blood pressure

- Help to manage the nausea and pain associated with chemotherapy treatments

- Eliminate the pain and fatigue of migraines

- Eliminate the symptoms of asthma and reduce asthma attacks

- Successfully treat including warts, psoriasis and atopic dermatitis

- Manage joint and muscle pain associate with chronic conditions like Fibromyalgia and Arthritis

- Eliminate sleep disorders like insomnia and manage the symptoms of sleep disorders like apnea

- Help treat obesity

The ADHD and ADD Guide for Parents
• Help treat children with ADD and ADHD

Eliminate the effects of severe stress and stress-related illness on the body

Why Let the Professionals Do It?

Making the decision to see a hypnotherapist or to use self-hypnosis can be a tough one depending on what condition you are using hypnosis to treat. For some conditions, like stress related illnesses, using self-hypnosis can be just as effective as seeing a hypnotherapist and can save you a lot of money since hypnosis treatments are usually not covered by insurance. But some conditions, especially those with a serious psychological cause, really need the expertise of a trained psychologist that also knows hypnosis.

In order to be able to make the best decision about what type of treatment is right for you it's important that you be honest about your skills at self-hypnosis. If you are just learning self-hypnosis or if you've never done self-hypnosis before then you should probably see a trained hypnotherapist for at least a few sessions just to see well you respond to hypnosis. If you feel that the hypnosis treatments are effective then you can start learning how to use self-hypnosis. Millions of people successfully use self-hypnosis every day in order to deal with anxieties, phobias, cravings and other problems.

Some New Age hypnotists believe that really all hypnosis is self-hypnosis since even the suggestions of the hypnotist won't be effective unless your mind is relaxed and receptive to them. There is an entire sect of hypnotists that believe the job of the hypnotherapist is just to assist you as you hypnotize and heal yourself. If you are very open to hypnosis and you can put yourself into a state of increased awareness and concentration while your body and mind are totally relaxed then you might do very well using self-hypnosis. But you should still see a hypnotherapist at least once so that you know how you respond to a hypnotherapy session run by a professional.

The underlying principle of hypnosis is that the patient wants to change. If you don't want to change the behavior or the condition that you're seeking hypnosis for then it won't matter if you are seeing a hypnotherapist with an extensive background in psychology, a New Age practitioner that is certified to treat addictions and other related problems with hypnosis, or self-hypnotizing to try and change your own behavior patterns. The success or failure of the hypnosis treatment lies entirely in whether or not you really, deep down, want to change.

If you really do want to make a change in your behavior or help your body fight off a medical condition then you will see some type of success with hypnosis. How much success is entirely up to you. Even if you choose to see a trained hypnotherapist on a regular basis you should consider using self-hypnosis as a treatment at home to boost your success and to keep progressing in your recovery.

Chapter 6- Training Children with ADHD/ADD for Success

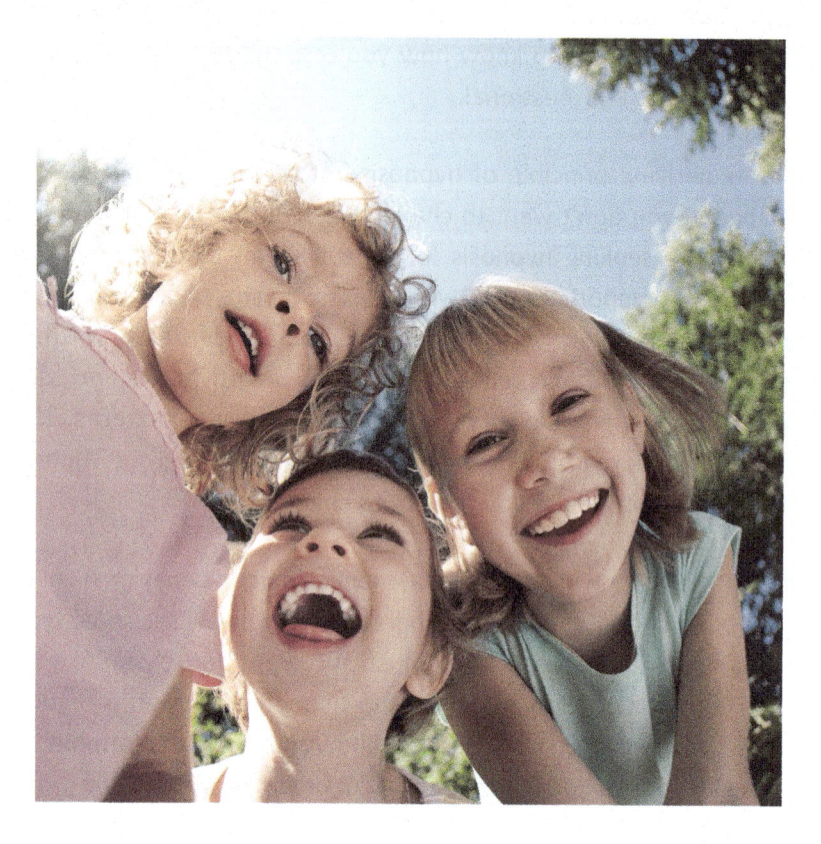

A lot of grownups with ADD perceive themselves constantly weighed down with everyday life. This means that they in general wake up feeling like they are behind the schedule on all the things they have to do, use up the entire day on high speed so as to get all those things completed, and yet still go to bed nearly all nights feeling like they never got anyplace. Or, they use up the entire day in a fog, continuously conscious of all the things on that to-do list, but never gathering together up the enthusiasm to engage in the tasks. This leaves them feeling disorganized, uncreative, discontented, lethargic, at fault ...and the list goes on.

Rose McCloud
Here are 8 important abilities for handling ADD.

1. Slow Down

ADDers appear to be for all time working on a hyper drive star...mentally, physically, or both. In my view, slowing down when you feel hurried, stressed out, weighed down, etc. is the first and most essential ability for handling ADD.

2. Put into Practice Superb Self-Care

ADDers have a tendency to put themselves at the end. Why is it so? How will you ever "get it together" if you do not set aside time and energy for yourself?

3. Know Your Own ADD

ADD has an effect on us all in diverse ways. You cannot efficiently handle ADD without being conscious of the particular manner in which it has an effect on you, and the particular manner in which your problems are set off.

4. Keenly Use Your Learning and Processing Methods

Categorizing the natural methods in which you are able to carry on concentrating and processing information and feelings will make your personal and professional lives much simpler.

5. Concentrate on Your Strengths

Everybody has strong points, expertise, aptitudes, and fervors. Increasing the time you use up on these good things will add to both your sense of worth and your contentment.

6. Think Optimistically

Process of pessimistic thinking can be overturned. Pessimistic thinking will hold you back. Optimistic thinking will boost you ahead.

7. Plan the Time to Plan…Everything

Planning does not all the time come effortlessly to ADDers. Developing tools and methods for planning will make more efficient the administration and time managing, but you have to take it one step ahead and plan the time to make use of them.

8. Take Challenges

This does not turn to speed racing or skydiving! It suggests to stepping out of your comfort region and doing things that may not be comfortable, like request for that increment, taking up that new pastime, or practicing that lifelong fervor. If you do not take the challenge, you will not get the return.

Plan Ahead the Daily Activities When They Reach Adulthood

Details seem to be useless to those adults who are suffering from Attention Deficit Disorder (ADD). We do have our goals clear in our minds, and cannot wait to have it achieved, hoping that there was some way to skip all the work required to be done in the process. Sadly enough, this attitude tends to get us overwhelmed, when we are to start the project. We seem to know what we want at the end, without having any idea of what needs to be done at the beginning.

This story is true for the everyday life as well. Adults suffering from ADD, generally start their day being sure of their goals, but they can't seem to get their priorities right and decide where to start from. This causes them to feel stressed and guilty, which makes them feel bad, and ultimately work less.

To avoid such a situation, these adults should develop the habit of making a daily planning routine.

In order to develop such a routine, the following 3 steps can be practiced:

1. Deciding On a Time to Do the Planning

The time of the day when the planning process can be done should be decided first. This should require only about 15 minutes, and the time could either be set specifically (say 8:00 PM) or could just be something like the time "right before bed."

The time late in the day is usually most preferred by the adults with ADD, since that is when they are the most alert. This is helpful since it allows one to plan for the next day, instead of worrying over it when they should go to bed!

2. Reviewing the To-Do List

Firstly make sure that you do use a to-do list, (if you don't then make one). This can be reviewed during each of your planning sessions, to remind you of what needs to be done. It also helps you feel good about all that you have already done during the day.

You must regularly re-write the list, deleting all the completed tasks and adding the new ones. The most urgent and important of the tasks should be noted at the top of the list. You may break the large ones into 3-5 steps, noting it down on your list.

The ADHD and ADD Guide for Parents

3. Reviewing the Calendar

Now, go through your daily planner (assuming that you are now finally using one!). Check your next day's appointments and block off those times on the planner, not forgetting the travel time. Now you can plan how to set aside some of your remaining time for the jobs on the to-do list.

Thus, spending just 15 minutes on planning the schedule can take away the everyday stress from the life of an adult with ADD, and can help one move ahead.

Setting Your Child Up for Job Success

For a lot of people with ADD, work life can be complex. If your operational surroundings are not ADD responsive, then you may well find yourself feeling constantly disordered and hassled out at work. Whether or not you decide to give out information about your analysis with your employer, the subsequent approaches can aid you become more efficient at work.

1. Look for a Profession that you are Zealous About:

People with ADD have the most accomplishment when doing something that they are fervently involved in. If you are in a profession or a job that you are not zealous about, odds are your ADD problems will exhibit themselves. The best way to keep away from this is to come across a job that you in fact take pleasure in and have faith in.

2. Build up Structure:

It is not unknown that ADDers work well with structure. If your job is short of structure, generate some.

If you are self-employed, make up a timetable for yourself. Decide on what your working days will be, and what your days off will be. And abide them. In addition, plan out particular working hours for yourself.

If another person or company employs you, ask for particular time limits on projects you are handed over. In addition, you can ask for a weekly meeting with your manager in which you bring him or her up to date on all the things you have been doing. This will let YOU to go through your development and stay conscious of all the jobs that you are coping with.

3. Pass on the Details:

I have on no account met an ADDer who takes pleasure in working with particulars. In general, people with ADD are the problem solvers, the innovative, and the organizers. A good number of ADDers will be exceptionally efficient when working with these stimulating and tricky features of the work, and a lot less efficient when working with executive job.

If you are self-employed, take on an associate - even though you think you cannot manage to pay for it. Visualize how much more efficient - and beneficial - you may well be if you did not have to be bothered about rules and regulations.

If another person or company employs you, pass on work to executive associates and any person whom you deal with. If there is no one for you to pass on to, give explanation to your manager that you work best when you do not have to be slowed down with executive jobs. Draw attention to all your expertise, strong points, and achievements. Let your manager know that you may possibly be giving in even more if you had some body to lend a hand with the particulars.

The ADHD and ADD Guide for Parents

4. Plan the Time to Plan:

It is not sufficient to plan your day, you must also think out the time to plan. Prior to your leaving work at the end of the day, use up 15 minutes to have a look at your to do list. See what you completed and what yet has to be done and up to date the list. In addition use this time to up to date your calendars, and fragment exceptional projects into steps. Using up the time to do this each work day will have you feeling more on top of things, and will also help you out to switch over out of work time and into personal time.

5. Get Over Fastidiousness:

Fastidiousness puts off growth. If you come across something that may well be enhanced every time you have a look at a paper or a report, it will never get off your table. There is a big distinction between "a good job" and "a perfect job." "A good job" is job done well; "a perfect job" does not happen. Nothing in this planet is just the right thing, so do yourself a big help and forget about it.

CHAPTER 7- WHAT'S IT LIKE LIVING WITH ADHD/ADD?

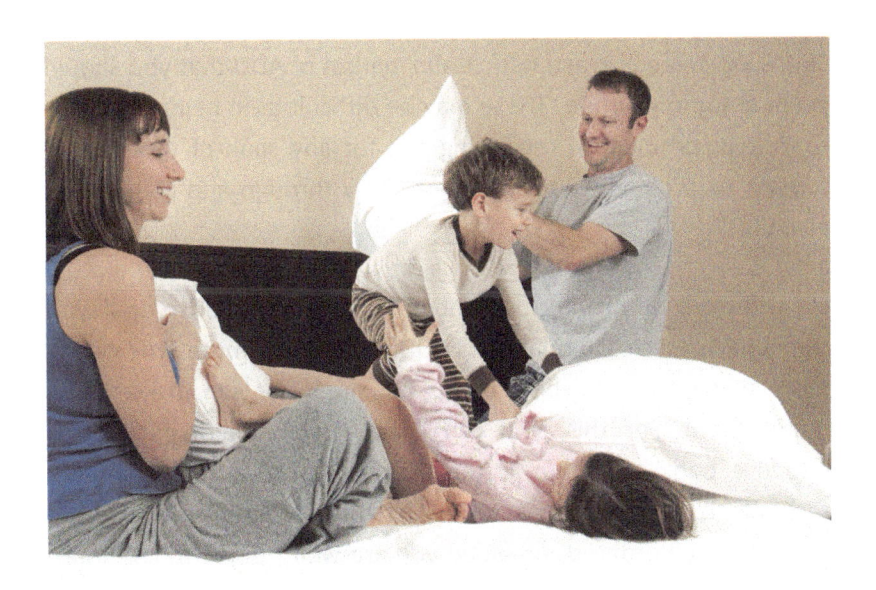

Life ahead may be easy for a child, a teenager, or even an adult diagnosed with ADD. For somebody, just diagnosed with ADD, predicting the life in future might not be easy, as one may not know how the symptoms would continue to remain and how the problem would be affected by age. However, thankfully, as time moves on, one starts to understand how to deal with ADD more efficiently, so that it causes fewer troubles in life.

Children with ADD are usually unmindful, reckless, or may get distracted easily or may show too much of goings-on. Also, the symptoms remain mostly the same even in other age groups. However, dealing with these symptoms does improve significantly, as one gets older.

The affect ADD can have on your life is largely determined by the medication you choose for treating the disorder. You may wish to consult the doctor to give you an advice on the future effects of

The ADHD and ADD Guide for Parents

taking stimulants, and also the implications of other medicines. Medicines are useful in dealing with ADD, though you can also try a behavior therapy too.

There are some characteristic traits, typical of ADD that you should prepare for in your life. These may be difficulties in being attentive to details, problem in remaining still for any span of time, being fidgety, or problem in being able to stay through and complete a given task.

Nevertheless, you can do a number of things in order to deal with the behavior typically related to ADD. To become more orderly and more managed in keeping things, an organizer can prove to be quite useful. For this, you can choose from anything like the effective book calendars to the digital organizers that are quite technologically sophisticated, to personal assistants. These will keep you well ordered, provided you are well trained to use these devices so that they can remember your important information and schedules.

These routines and schedules should be used to their maximum. You will naturally be inclined to forget and be careless. So by using a proper device you will tend to behave more unlike your nature and thus make lesser mistakes. So, it is always better to use automation.

You may also wish to be a part of groups, for support, or may at least want the company of the ones like you. You may feel the need for someone to confide in, who can understand you situation well. A person with ADD could be a perfect companion since they may be able to connect with you better than any friend or a family member, since they can support you only to a limit.

Rose McCloud
What Can Parents Do?

With the diagnosis of your child with Attention Deficit Disorder, you may feel a shower of emotions: remorse, a feeling of not being in charge, or comfort for now being aware of your child's problem, or frustration. However in the midst of all this turmoil, do not forget that your child's situation is not out of control. There are a number of ways in which you can help your child use his talents, and deal with ADD.

The first most important step is to properly do your research and know everything about ADD. You would thus be in a better position to help your child, and understand the problems. You would also become more aware of the popular treatments, and be more prepared to face what might come next. It should also be helpful in preparing you to work with the doctor for managing the disorder successfully.

With the advice of your doctor, you should also plan whether you should get your child medicated. This depends on your individual opinion and the decision is entirely personal. According to some parents, being able to provide their children with means to lead a normal life is the best opportunity that they can give. But, for others, medication is not a good choice. However, no matter what you decide, you should be sure of it and well informed about your choice.

In any case, even if you are using medication, some strategies of behavior therapies should be applied to help manage your child's actions. These prepare your child with lasting skills to provide them with help in becoming efficient and productive. The strategies for your child's actions and the consequences should be set by you. Children suffering from ADD need to have well defined limits set on their actions and must be treated with steady discipline.

The ADHD and ADD Guide for Parents
You should be your child's best supporter, and must encourage your child. Make sure that the way they are treated at school and at home, in such that it would guarantee you child's progress. You, along with the teachers and doctors, should be like a team whose target must be to assist your child in being successful.

So lend a hand and help your child grow to be a self-assured and joyful person. Recognize their potential and let them know to what extent you love them. A child diagnosed with ADD habitually goes through depression and low sense of worth. So if you see such cases arising then take necessary actions to steer clear of this outcome. And if the situation demands, request for expert help.

Joining a good support group and reaching out to people who share the same state of affairs, could be useful. Often the top suggestions you can get is from a person who has been through a similar situation. Make use of the experiences of life!

About The Author

Rose McCloud is a developmental pediatrician. She was born in Britain but was raised in Idaho by the American couple that adopted her.

Rose has always had the desire to treat children. She originally wanted to become a pediatrician but in medical school, she realized that she is much more effective in diagnosis and treating children with developmental problems.

Today, Rose is a wonderful mother to Theodore. Her husband was in the army but unfortunately died during his second tour in Iraq.